Ketogenic Air Fryer Recipes for Daily Healthy Meals

I0134875

Easy and Healthy Recipes to Make Unforgettable First Courses

Morgan Parry

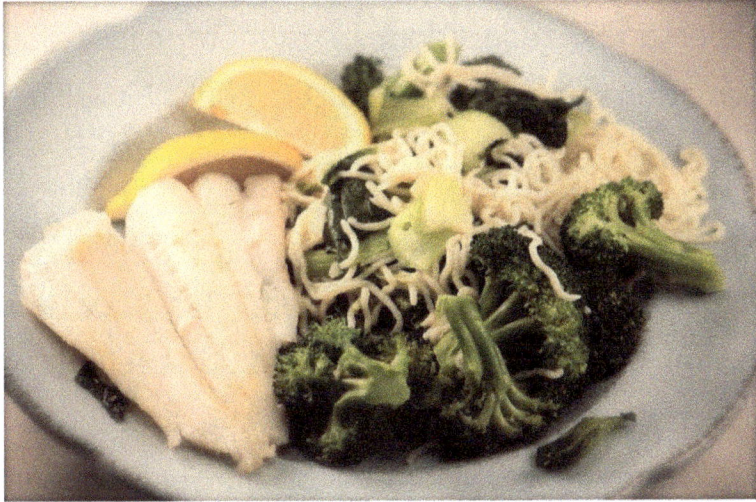

advice. The content within this book has been derived from various sources. Please consult a licensed professional before attempting any techniques outlined in this book.

By reading this document, the reader agrees that under no circumstances is the author responsible for any losses, direct or indirect, which are incurred as a result of the use of information contained within this document, including, but not limited to, — errors, omissions, or inaccuracies.

Table of Contents

Cheddar Biscuits

Prep time: 15 minutes

Cooking time: 8 minutes

Servings: 4

Ingredients:

- ½ cup almond flour

- ¼ cup Cheddar cheese, shredded

- ¾ teaspoon salt

- 1 egg, beaten

- 1 tablespoon mascarpone

- 1 tablespoon coconut oil, melted

- ¾ teaspoon baking powder

- ½ teaspoon apple cider vinegar

- ¼ teaspoon ground nutmeg

Directions:

1.   In the big bowl mix up ground nutmeg, almond flour, salt, and baking powder. After this, add egg, apple

cider vinegar, coconut oil, and mascarpone. Add cheese and knead the soft dough. Then with the help of the fingertips make the small balls (biscuits). Preheat the air fryer to 400F. Then line the air fryer basket with parchment. Place the cheese biscuits on the parchment and cook them for 8 minutes at 400F. Shake the biscuits during the cooking to avoid burning. The cooked cheese biscuits will have a golden brown color.

Nutrition: calories 102, fat 9.1, fiber 0.4, carbs 1.6, protein 4.3

Eggplant Spread

Preparation time: 5 minutes

Cooking time: 20 minutes

Servings: 4

Ingredients:

• 3 eggplants

• Salt and black pepper to the taste 2 tablespoons chives, chopped

• 2 tablespoons olive oil

• 2 teaspoons sweet paprika

Directions:

1. Put the eggplants in your air fryer's basket and cook them for 20 minutes at 380 degrees F. Peel the eggplants, put them in a blender, add the rest of the ingredients, pulse well, divide into bowls and serve for breakfast.

Nutrition: calories 190, fat 7, fiber 3, carbs 5, protein 3

Fish Sticks

Prep time: 15 minutes

Cooking time: 10 minutes

Servings: 4

Ingredients:

- 8 oz cod fillet
- 1 egg, beaten
- ¼ cup coconut flour
- ¼ teaspoon ground coriander
- ¼ teaspoon ground paprika
- ¼ teaspoon ground cumin
- ¼ teaspoon Pink salt
- 1/3 cup coconut flakes
- 1 tablespoon mascarpone
- 1 teaspoon heavy cream
- Cooking spray

Directions:

1.   Chop the cod fillet roughly and put it in the blender. Add egg, coconut flour ground coriander, paprika, cumin, salt, and blend the mixture until smooth. After this, transfer it in the bowl. Line the chopping board with parchment. Place the fish mixture over the parchment and flatten it in the shape of the flat square. Then cut the fish square into sticks. In the separated bowl whisk together heavy cream and mascarpone. Sprinkle every fish stick with mascarpone mixture and after this, coat in the coconut flakes. Preheat the air fryer to 400F. Spray the air fryer basket with cooking spray and arrange the fish sticks inside. Cook the fish sticks for 10 minutes. Flip them on another side in halfway of cooking.

Nutrition: calories 101, fat 5, fiber 1, carbs 1.9, protein 12.4

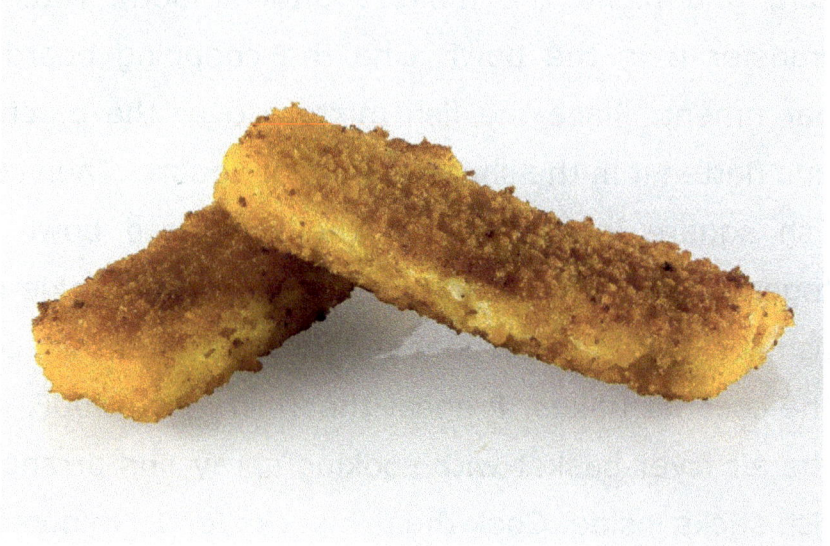

Sprouts Hash

Preparation time: 5 minutes

Cooking time: 20 minutes

Servings: 4

Ingredients:

- 1 tablespoon olive oil

- 1 pound Brussels sprouts, shredded 4 eggs, whisked

- ½ cup coconut cream

- Salt and black pepper to the taste 1 tablespoon chives, chopped

- ¼ cup cheddar cheese, shredded

Directions:

1. Preheat the Air Fryer at 360 degrees F and grease it with the oil. Spread the Brussels sprouts on the bottom of the fryer, then add the eggs mixed with the rest of the ingredients, toss a bit and cook for 20 minutes. Divide between plates and serve.

Nutrition: calories 242, fat 12, fiber 3, carbs 5, protein 9

Fried Bacon

Prep time: 10 minutes

Cooking time: 12 minutes

Servings: 4

Ingredients:

- 10 oz bacon

- 3 oz pork rinds

- 2 eggs, beaten

- ½ teaspoon salt

- ½ teaspoon ground black pepper

- Cooking spray

Directions:

1.	Cut the bacon into 4 cubes and sprinkle with salt and ground black pepper. After this dip the bacon cubes in the beaten eggs and coat in the pork rinds. Preheat the air fryer to 395F. Spray the air fryer basket with cooking spray and put the bacon cubes inside. Cook them for 6 minutes. Then flip the bacon on another side and cook for 6 minutes more or until it is light brown.

Salmon Salad

Preparation time: 5 minutes

Cooking time: 8 minutes

Servings: 4

Ingredients:

- 4 salmon fillets, boneless 2 tablespoons olive oil

- Salt and black pepper to the taste 3 cups kale leaves, shredded

- 2 teaspoons balsamic vinegar

Directions:

1. Put the fish in your air fryer's basket, season with salt and pepper, drizzle half of the oil over them, cook at 400 degrees F for 4 minutes on each side, cool down and cut into medium cubes. In a bowl, mix the kale with salt, pepper, vinegar, the rest of the oil and the salmon, toss gently and serve for lunch.

Nutrition: calories 240, fat 14, fiber 3, carbs 5, protein 10

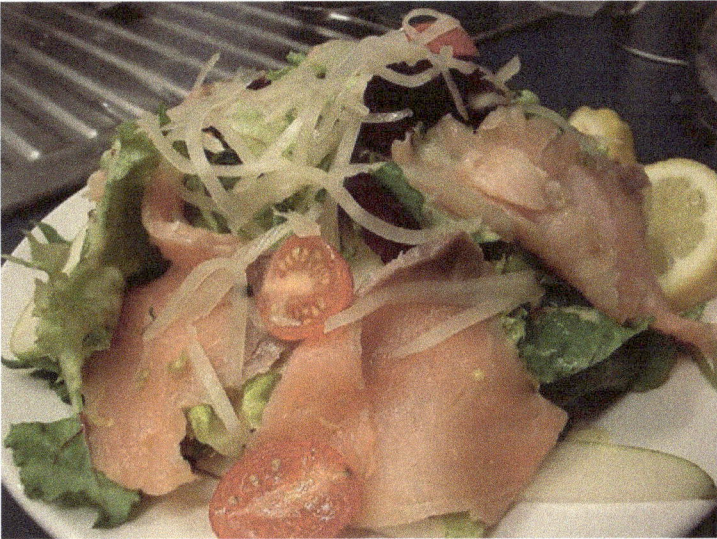

Zucchini Pasta

Prep time: 15 minutes

Cooking time: 14 minutes

Servings: 4

Ingredients:

- ½ cup ground beef

- ¼ teaspoon salt

- ½ teaspoon chili flakes

- ¼ teaspoon dried dill

- 2 zucchinis, trimmed

- 2 tablespoons mascarpone

- 1 teaspoon olive oil

- ½ teaspoon ground black pepper

- Cooking spray

Directions:

1.   In the mixing bowl mix up ground beef, salt, chili flakes, and dill. Then make the small meatballs. Preheat

the air fryer to 365F. Spray the air fryer basket with cooking spray and place the meatballs inside in one layer.

2. Cook the meatballs for 12 minutes. Shake them after 6 minutes of cooking to avoid burning. Then remove the meatballs from the air fryer. With the help of the spiralizer make the zucchini noodles and sprinkle them with olive oil and ground black pepper. Place the zucchini noodles in the air fryer and cook them for 2 minutes at 400F. Then mix up zucchini noodles and mascarpone and transfer them in the serving plates. Top the noodles with cooked meatballs.

Nutrition: calories 145, fat 8.8, fiber 2.3, carbs 7.5, protein 10.7

Paprika Turkey Mix

Preparation time: 5 minutes

Cooking time: 20 minutes

Servings: 4

Ingredients:

- turkey breast, boneless, skinless and cubed 2 teaspoons olive oil

- ½ teaspoon sweet paprika

- Salt and black pepper to the taste 2 cups bok choy, torn and steamed 1 tablespoon balsamic vinegar

Directions:

1. In a bowl, mix the turkey with the oil, paprika, salt and pepper, toss, transfer them to your Air Fryer's basket and cook at 350 degrees F for 20 minutes. In a salad, mix the turkey with all the other ingredients, toss and serve for lunch.

Nutrition: calories 250, fat 13, fiber 3, carbs 6, protein 14

Spiced Salmon and Cilantro Croquettes

Prep time: 10 minutes

Cooking time: 8 minutes

Servings: 4

Ingredients:

- 1-pound smoked salmon, boneless and flaked

- 1 egg, beaten

- 1 tablespoon almond flour

- ½ teaspoon ground black pepper

- ¼ teaspoon ground cumin

- ½ teaspoon ground nutmeg

- 1 tablespoon fresh cilantro, chopped

- 1 teaspoon avocado oil

Directions:

1.   Put the salmon in the bowl and churn it with the help of the fork until you get the smooth mass. Then add an egg, almond flour, ground black pepper, cumin,

nutmeg, and cilantro. Stir the ingredients until they are smooth. Preheat the air fryer to 365F. Wet your hands and make the croquettes. Then place them in the air fryer in one layer and sprinkle with avocado oil. Cook the croquettes for 5 minutes. Then flip them on another side and cook for 3 minutes more.

Nutrition: calories 210, fat 11.9, fiber 1, carbs 2, protein 25

Oregano Cod and Arugula Mix

Preparation time: 5 minutes

Cooking time: 12 minutes

Servings: 4

Ingredients:

- tablespoons fresh cilantro, minced
- pound cod fillets, boneless, skinless and cubed 1 spring onion, chopped
- Salt and black pepper to the taste
- ½ teaspoon sweet paprika
- ½ teaspoon oregano, ground A drizzle of olive oil
- cups baby arugula

Directions:

1.   In a bowl, mix the cod with salt, pepper, paprika, oregano and the oil, toss, transfer the cubes to your air fryer's basket and cook at 360 degrees F for 12 minutes. In a salad bowl, mix the cod with the remaining ingredients, toss, divide between plates and serve.

Nutrition: calories 240, fat 11, fiber 3, carbs 5, protein 8

Shrimp Salad

Prep time: 15 minutes

Cooking time: 3 minutes

Servings: 4

Ingredients:

- 1-pound shrimps, peeled

- 1 tablespoon lemon juice

- ½ teaspoon ground cardamom

- ¼ teaspoon salt

- ½ teaspoon ground paprika

- 1 tablespoon olive oil

- 1 garlic clove, diced

- 1 avocado, peeled, pitted, chopped

- 1 teaspoon chives, chopped

Directions:

1.   Put the shrimps in the big bowl. Add lemon juice, ground nutmeg, salt, and ground paprika. Mix up the

shrimps and leave them for 10 minutes to marinate. Meanwhile, preheat the air fryer to 400F. Put the marinated shrimps in the air fryer and cook them for 3 minutes. It is recommended to arrange shrimps in one layer. Meanwhile, put the chopped avocado in the bowl and sprinkle it with diced garlic and chives. Cool the shrimps to the room temperature and add in the avocado bowl. Sprinkle the salad with olive oil. After this, gently mix the salad with the help of two spoons.

Nutrition: calories 271, fat 15.3, fiber 3.6, carbs 6.7, protein 26.9

Pork and Zucchinis

Preparation time: 5 minutes

Cooking time: 30 minutes

Servings: 4

Ingredients:

- 2 pounds pork stew meat, cubed 2 zucchinis, cubed

- Salt and black pepper to the taste

- ½ cup beef stock

- ½ teaspoon smoked paprika A handful cilantro, chopped

Directions:

1. In a pan that fits your air fryer, mix all the ingredients, toss, introduce in your air fryer and cook at 370 degrees F for 30 minutes. Divide into bowls and serve right away.

Nutrition: calories 245, fat 12, fiber 2, carbs 5, protein 14

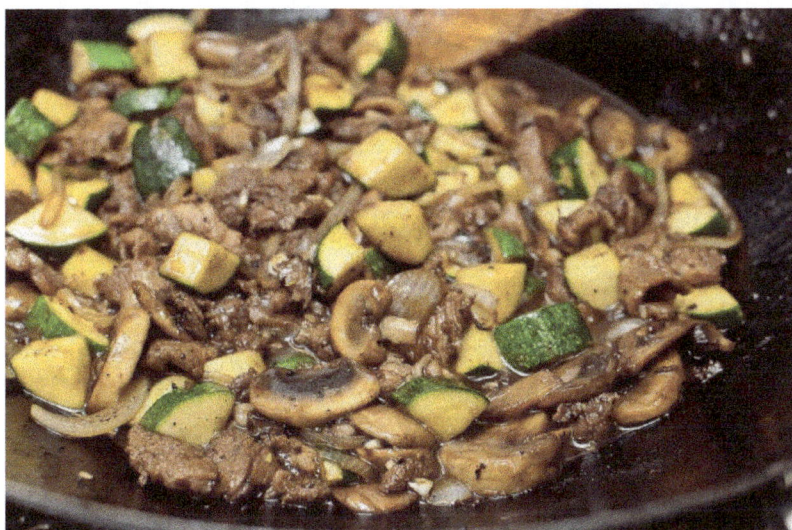

Rosemary Salmon

Prep time: 10 minutes

Cooking time: 7 minutes

Servings: 2

Ingredients:

- 4 oz Feta cheese, sliced

- 1 lemon slice, chopped

- ½ teaspoon dried rosemary

- 1 teaspoon apple cider vinegar

- ½ teaspoon ground paprika

- 1-pound salmon fillet

- 1 teaspoon olive oil

- ½ teaspoon salt

- Cooking spray

Directions:

1. Rub the salmon with dried rosemary and salt. Then sprinkle the fish with ground paprika and apple cider

vinegar. Preheat the air fryer to 395F. Line the air fryer basket with baking paper and put the salmon fillet on it. Spray it with cooking spray and cook for 3 minutes. Then flip the salmon on another side and cook it for 4 minutes more. After this, cut the cooked salmon into 2 servings and put it on the serving plate. Top the fish with sliced feta and chopped lemon slice. Sprinkle the meal with the olive oil before serving.

Nutrition: calories 596, fat 45, fiber 0.4, carbs 1.2, protein 47.4

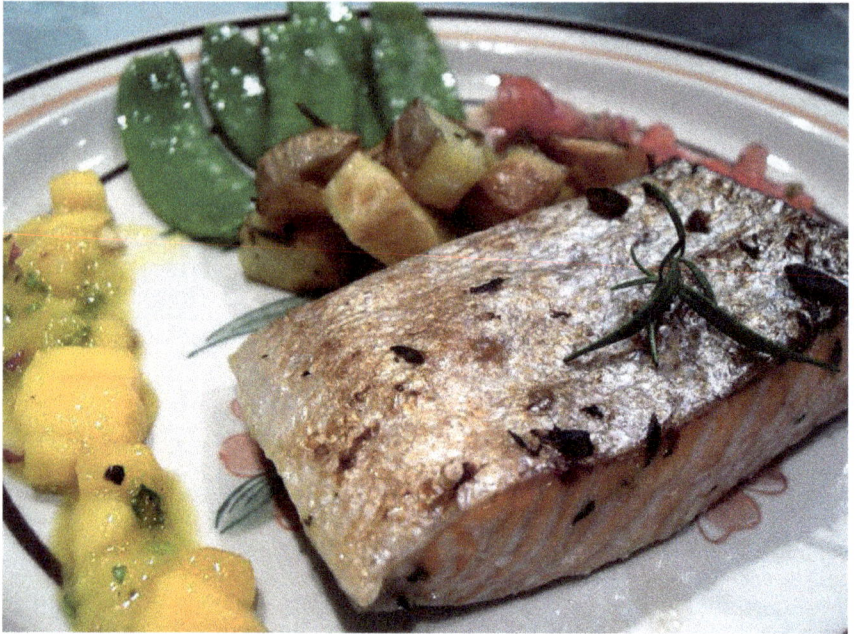

Seafood Bowls

Preparation time: 5 minutes

Cooking time: 12 minutes

Servings: 4

Ingredients:

• 2 salmon fillets, boneless, skinless and cubed 8 ounces shrimp, peeled and deveined

• Salt and black pepper to the taste 5 garlic cloves, minced

• teaspoon sweet paprika 2 tablespoons olive oil

Directions:

1. In a pan that fits the air fryer, combine all the ingredients, toss, cover and cook at 370 degrees F for 12 minutes. Divide into bowls and serve for lunch.

Nutrition: calories 270, fat 8, fiber 2, carbs 4, protein 7

Beef Chili

Prep time: 15 minutes

Cooking time: 29 minutes

Servings: 4

Ingredients:

- 2 spring onions, chopped

- 2 medium green bell peppers, chopped

- 1 tablespoon avocado oil

- ½ teaspoon salt

- ½ teaspoon ground black pepper

- 2 cups ground beef

- 1 teaspoon ground paprika

- 1 teaspoon chili flakes

- ½ teaspoon white pepper

- 1 teaspoon ground cumin

- ½ teaspoon ground coriander

- 1 chili pepper, chopped

- 1 cup beef broth

- 1 tablespoon keto tomato sauce

- 1 cup lettuce leaves

Directions:

1.   Put the spring onions in the air fryer pan. Add green bell peppers, avocado oil, salt, and ground black pepper. Stir the mixture gently. Preheat the air fryer to 365F and place the pan with vegetables inside. Cook them for 4 minutes. Then stir well. In the mixing bowl mix up ground beef, ground paprika, chili flakes, white pepper, ground cumin, ground coriander, and tomato sauce Put the meat mixture over the vegetables and carefully stir it with the help of the spoon. Add chili pepper and beef broth. Stir the chili gently. Cook it at 365F for 25 minutes. Stir the chili every 5 minutes of cooking. When the chili is cooked, cool it for 5-10 minutes. Then fill the lettuce leaves with chili and transfer in the serving plates.

Nutrition: calories 177, fat 9.3, fiber 2.4, carbs 7.7, protein 15.5

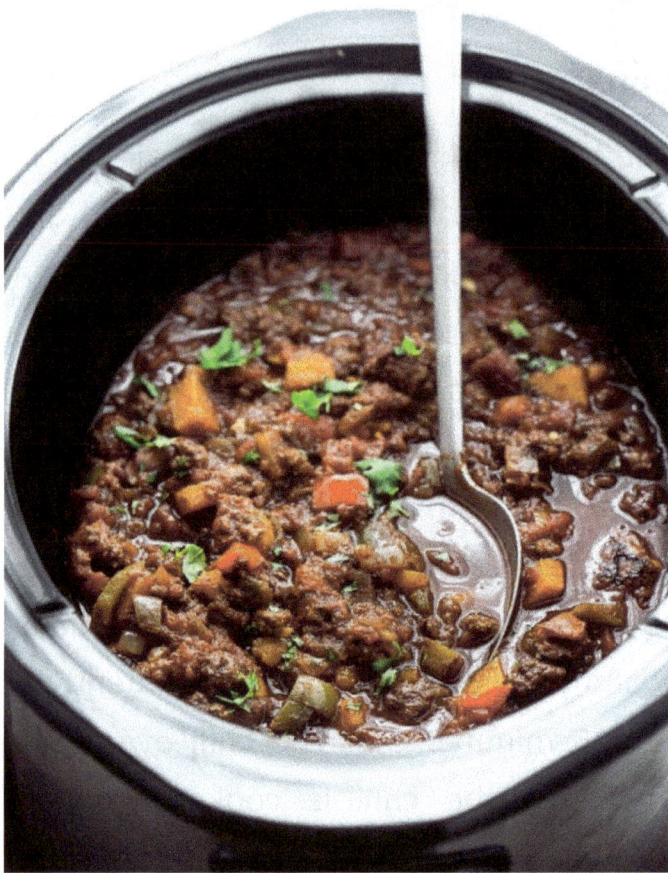

Eggplant Bowls

Preparation time: 5 minutes

Cooking time: 15 minutes

Servings: 4

Ingredients:

- cups eggplants, cubed 1 cup keto tomato sauce 1 teaspoon olive oil

- 1 cup mozzarella, shredded

Directions:

- In a pan that fits the air fryer, combine all the ingredients except the mozzarella and toss. Sprinkle the cheese on top, introduce the pan in the machine and cook at 390 degrees F for 15 minutes. Divide between plates and serve for lunch.

Nutrition: calories 220, fat 9, fiber 2, carbs 6, protein 9

Chicken Rolls

Prep time: 15 minutes

Cooking time: 18 minutes

Servings: 4

Ingredients:

- 2 large zucchini

- ½ cup Cheddar cheese, shredded

- 1-pound chicken breast, skinless, boneless

- 1 teaspoon dried oregano

- ½ teaspoon olive oil

- 1 teaspoon salt

- 2 spring onions, chopped

- 1 teaspoon ground paprika

- ½ teaspoon ground turmeric

- ½ cup keto tomato sauce

Directions:

1.   Preheat the skillet well and pour the olive oil inside. Put the onions in it and sprinkle with salt, ground paprika, and ground turmeric. Cook the onion for 5 minutes over the medium-high heat. Stir it from time to time. Meanwhile, shred the chicken. Add it in the skillet. Then add oregano. Stir well and cook the mixture for 2 minutes. After this, remove the skillet from the heat. Cut the zucchini into halves (lengthwise). Then make the zucchini slices with the help of the vegetable peeler. Put 3 zucchini slices on the chopping board overlapping each of them. Then spread the surface of them with the shredded chicken mixture. Roll the zucchini carefully in the shape of the roll. Repeat the same steps with remaining zucchini and shredded chicken mixture. Line the air fryer pan with parchment and put the enchilada rolls inside. Sprinkle them with tomato sauce Preheat the air fryer to 350F. Top the zucchini rolls (enchiladas) with Cheddar cheese and put in the air fryer basket. Cook the meal for 10 minutes.

Nutrition: calories 245, fat 9.3, fiber 3, carbs 10.3, protein 29.9

Chicken and Asparagus

Preparation time: 5 minutes

Cooking time: 20 minutes

Servings: 4

Ingredients:

• 4 chicken breasts, skinless, boneless and halved 1 tablespoon sweet paprika

• bunch asparagus, trimmed and halved 1 tablespoon olive oil

• Salt and black pepper to the taste

Directions:

1. In a bowl, mix all the ingredients, toss, put them in your Air Fryer's basket and cook at 390 degrees F for 20 minutes. Divide between plates and serve for lunch.

Nutrition: calories 230, fat 11, fiber 3, carbs 5, protein 12

Cheesy Calzone

Prep time: 15 minutes

Cooking time: 8 minutes

Servings: 2

Ingredients:

- 2 tablespoons almond flour
- 2 tablespoons flax meal
- 1 tablespoon coconut oil, softened
- ¼ teaspoon salt
- ¼ teaspoon baking powder
- 2 ham slices, chopped
- 1 oz Parmesan, grated
- 1 egg yolk, whisked
- 1 tablespoon spinach, chopped
- Cooking spray

Directions:

1.   Make calzone dough: mix up almond flour, flax meal, coconut oil, salt, and baking powder. Knead the dough until soft and smooth. Then roll it up with the help of the rolling pin and cut into halves. Fill every dough half with chopped ham, grated Parmesan, and spinach. Fold the dough in the shape of calzones and secure the edges. Then brush calzones with the whisked egg yolk. Preheat the air fryer basket to 350F. Place the calzones in the air fryer basket and spray them with cooking spray. Cook them for 8 minutes or until they are light brown. Flip the calzones on another side after 4 minutes of cooking.

Nutrition: calories 368, fat 31, fiber 5.4, carbs 10.2, protein 18.1

Cilantro Turkey Casserole

Preparation time: 5 minutes

Cooking time: 25 minutes

Servings: 4

Ingredients:

- tablespoons butter, melted 12 ounces cream cheese, soft

- 2 cups turkey breasts, skinless, boneless and cut into strips 1 cups zucchinis, sliced

- 2 teaspoons sweet paprika

- 6 ounces cheddar cheese, grated

- ¼ cup cilantro, chopped

- Salt and black pepper to the taste

Directions:

1. In a baking dish that fits your air fryer, mix the butter with turkey, cream cheese and all the other ingredients except the cheddar cheese. Sprinkle the cheddar on top, put the dish in your air fryer and cook at

360 degrees F for 25 minutes. Divide between plates and serve for lunch.

Nutrition: calories 280, fat 10, fiber 2, carbs 4, protein 12

Dill Egg Salad

Prep time: 10 minutes

Cooking time: 17 minutes

Servings: 3

Ingredients:

- 1 avocado, peeled, pitted

- 5 eggs

- 1 tablespoon ricotta cheese

- 1 tablespoon heavy cream

- 1 teaspoon mascarpone cheese

- ½ teaspoon minced garlic

- 1 pickled cucumber

- 1 tablespoon fresh dill, chopped

Directions:

1. Put the eggs in the air fryer basket and cook them for 17 minutes at 250F. Meanwhile, cut the avocado into

cubes and put them in the salad bowl. In the shallow bowl whisk together ricotta cheese, mascarpone, and minced garlic. Grate the pickled cucumber and add it in the cheese mixture. Add dill and stir the mixture well. When the eggs are cooked, cool them in the ice water and peel. Cut the eggs into the cubes and add in the avocado.

2.   Add cheese mixture and stir the salad well.

Nutrition: calories 275, fat 22.9, fiber 4.9, carbs 8.1, protein 11.7

Coconut Chicken

Preparation time: 4 minutes

Cooking time: 20 minutes

Servings: 4

Ingredients:

• 4 chicken breasts, skinless, boneless and cubed
Salt and black pepper to the taste

• ¼ cup coconut cream 1 teaspoon olive oil

• and ½ teaspoon sweet paprika

Directions:

1. Grease a pan that fits your air fryer with the oil, mix all the ingredients inside, introduce the pan in the fryer and cook at 370 degrees F for 17 minutes. Divide between plates and serve for lunch.

Nutrition: calories 250, fat 12, fiber 2, carbs 5, protein 11

Radish and Tuna Salad

Prep time: 15 minutes

Cooking time: 8 minutes

Servings: 2

Ingredients:

- ½ cup radish sprouts

- 8 oz tuna, smoked, boneless and shredded

- 1 egg, beaten

- 1 tablespoon coconut flour

- ½ teaspoon ground coriander

- ½ teaspoon lemon zest, grated

- 1 tablespoon olive oil

- ½ teaspoon salt

- 1 tablespoon lemon juice

- ½ cup radish, sliced

Directions:

1.   Mix up the tuna with coconut flour, ground coriander, lemon zest, and egg. Stir the mixture until homogenous. Preheat the air fryer to 400F. Then make the small tuna balls and put them in the hot air fryer. Sprinkle the tuna balls with ½ tablespoon of olive oil. Cook the tuna balls for 8 minutes. Flip the tuna balls on another side after 4 minutes of cooking.

2.   Meanwhile, mix up together radish sprouts and radish. Sprinkle the mixture with remaining olive oil, salt, and lemon juice. Shake it well. Then top the salad with tuna balls.

Nutrition: calories 342, fat 18.9, fiber 1.8, carbs 5.4, protein 35.7

Pork Bowls

Preparation time: 5 minutes

Cooking time: 20 minutes

Servings: 4

Ingredients:

- ½ pound pork stew meat, cubed

- ¼ cup keto tomato sauce 1 tablespoon olive oil

- cups mustard greens

- 1 yellow bell pepper, chopped 2 green onions, chopped

- Salt and black pepper to the taste

Directions:

1. In a pan that fits your air fryer, mix all the ingredients, toss, introduce the pan in the air fryer and cook at 370 degrees F for 20 minutes. Divide into bowls and serve for lunch.

Nutrition: calories 265, fat 12, fiber 3, carbs 5, protein 14

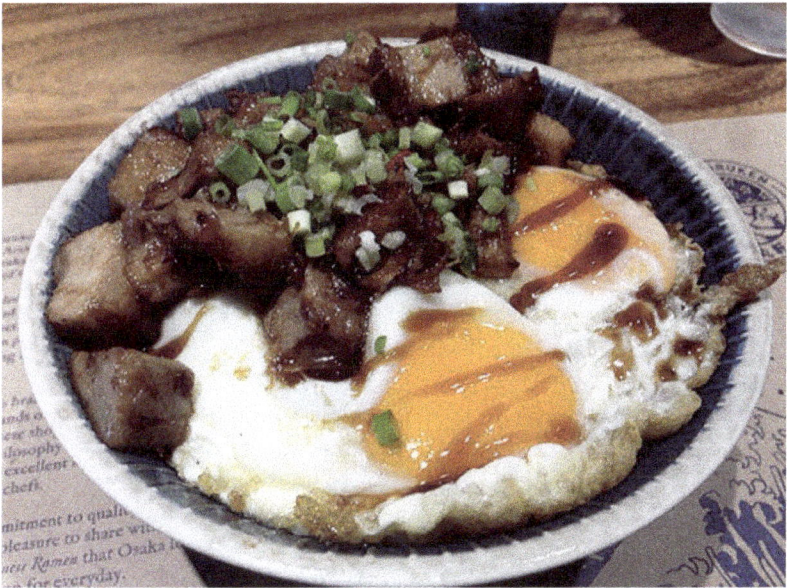

Broccoli Salad

Prep time: 10 minutes

Cooking time: 18 minutes

Servings: 2

Ingredients:

- 1 cup broccoli florets

- 1 teaspoon olive oil

- 1 tablespoon hazelnuts, chopped

- 4 bacon slices

- ½ teaspoon salt

- ½ teaspoon lemon zest, grated

- ½ teaspoon sesame oil

Directions:

1. Mix up broccoli florets with olive oil, salt, and lemon zest. Shake the vegetables well. Preheat the air fryer to 385F. Put the broccoli in the air fryer basket and cook for

8 minutes. Shake the broccoli after 4 minutes of cooking. Then transfer the broccoli in the salad bowl. Place the bacon in the air fryer and cook it at 400F for 10 minutes or until it is crunchy. Chop the cooked bacon and add in the broccoli. After this, add hazelnuts and sesame oil. Stir the salad gently.

Nutrition: calories 266, fat 20.9, fiber 1.4, carbs 4.1, protein 15.7

Chicken Stew

Preparation time: 5 minutes

Cooking time: 30 minutes

Servings: 6

Ingredients:

- tablespoon butter, soft 4 celery stalks, chopped
- red bell peppers, chopped
- 1 pound chicken breasts, skinless, boneless and cubed 2 teaspoons garlic, minced
- Salt and black pepper to the taste
- ½ cup coconut cream

Directions:

1. Grease a baking dish that fits your air fryer with the butter, add all the ingredients in the pan and toss them. Introduce the dish in the fryer, cook at 360 degrees F for 30 minutes, divide into bowls and serve for lunch.

Nutrition: calories 246, fat 12, fiber 2, carbs 6, protein 12

Chives Chicken

Prep time: 10 minutes

Cooking time: 12 minutes

Servings: 4

Ingredients:

- 4 chicken tenders

- ½ teaspoon ground paprika

- ½ teaspoon salt

- ½ cup coconut flakes

- 1 egg, beaten

- 1 tablespoon heavy cream

- ½ teaspoon dried dill

- ½ teaspoon onion powder

- 1 tablespoon chives, grinded

- 1 teaspoon sesame oil

Directions:

1.   Beat the chicken tenders gently with the help of the kitchen hammer. In the mixing bowl mix up salt, eggs heavy cream, dried dill, onion powder, and chives. Then dip the chicken tenders in the egg mixture and coat in the coconut flakes. Repeat the same steps one more time. Preheat the air fryer to 400F. Sprinkle the air fryer basket with sesame oil and place the chicken tenders inside. Cook the rack chicken for 6 minutes. Then flip it on another side and cook for 6 minutes more or until the chicken is light brown.

Nutrition: calories 354, fat 17.8, fiber 1.1, carbs 2.2, protein 44.2

Rosemary Zucchini Mix

Preparation time: 5 minutes

Cooking time: 12 minutes

Servings: 4

Ingredients:

- ¼ cup keto tomato sauce 1 tablespoon olive oil

- 8 zucchinis, roughly cubed

- Salt and black pepper to the taste

- ¼ teaspoon rosemary, dried

- ½ teaspoon basil, chopped

Directions:

1.   Grease a pan that fits your air fryer with the oil, add all the ingredients, toss, introduce the pan in the fryer and cook at 350 degrees F for 12 minutes. Divide into bowls and serve for lunch.

Nutrition: calories 200, fat 6, fiber 2, carbs 4, protein 6

Pork Casserole

Prep time: 15 minutes

Cooking time: 30 minutes

Servings: 6

Ingredients:

- 1 teaspoon taco seasonings

- 1 teaspoon sesame oil

- 1 teaspoon salt

- 2 cups ground pork

- ½ cup keto tomato sauce

- 2 low carb tortillas

- ½ cup Cheddar cheese, shredded

- ¼ cup mozzarella cheese, shredded

Directions:

1.   Chop the tortillas roughly. Brush the air fryer pan with sesame oil and place ½ part of chopped tortilla in it.

In the mixing bowl mix up taco seasonings, ground pork, and salt. Place ½ part of ground pork over the tortillas and top it with mozzarella cheese. Then cover the cheese with remaining tortillas, ground pork, and Cheddar cheese. Pour the marinara sauce over the cheese and cover the casserole with foil. Secure the edges. Preheat the air fryer to 395F. Put the casserole in the air fryer and cook it for 20 minutes. Then remove the foil and cook it for 10 minutes more.

Nutrition: calories 404, fat 27, fiber 2.9, carbs 7.4, protein 30.9

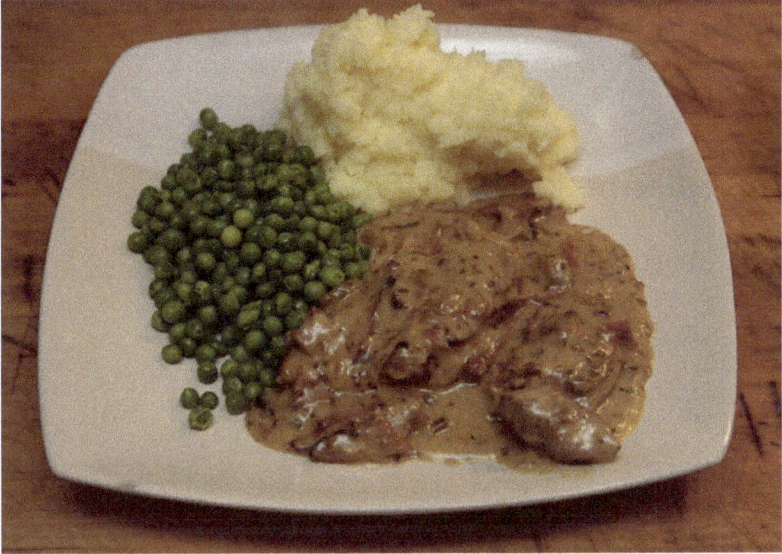

Kale Omelet

Preparation time: 10 minutes

Cooking time: 20 minutes **Servings:** 4

Ingredients:

- 1 eggplant, cubed

- 4 eggs, whisked

- 2 teaspoons cilantro, chopped Salt and black pepper to the taste

- ½ teaspoon Italian seasoning Cooking spray

- ½ cup kale, chopped

- 2 tablespoons cheddar, grated

- 2 tablespoons fresh basil, chopped

Directions:

1. In a bowl, mix all the ingredients except the cooking spray and whisk well. Grease a pan that fits your air fryer with the cooking spray, pour the eggs mix, spread, put the pan in the machine and cook at 370

degrees F for 20 minutes. Divide the mix between plates and serve for breakfast.

Nutrition: calories 241, fat 11, fiber 4, carbs 5, protein 12

Coconut Muffins

Prep time: 10 minutes

Cooking time: 10 minutes

Servings: 2

Ingredients:

- 1/3 cup almond flour

- 2 tablespoons Erythritol

- ¼ teaspoon baking powder

- 1 teaspoon apple cider vinegar

- 1 tablespoon coconut milk

- 1 tablespoon coconut oil, softened

- 1 teaspoon ground cinnamon

- Cooking spray

Directions:

1.   In the mixing bowl mix up almond flour. Erythritol, baking powder, and ground cinnamon. Add apple cider vinegar, coconut milk, and coconut oil. Stir the mixture

until smooth. Spray the muffin molds with cooking spray. Scoop the muffin batter in the muffin molds. Spray the surface of every muffin with the help of the spatula. Preheat the air fryer to 365F. Insert the rack in the air fryer. Place the muffins on the rack and cook them for 10 minutes at 365F. Then cool the cooked muffins well and remove them from the molds.

Nutrition: calories 107, fat 10.9, fiber 1.3, carbs 2.7, protein 1.2

Coconut Veggie and Eggs Bake

Preparation time: 5 minutes

Cooking time: 30 minutes

Servings: 6

Ingredients:

- Cooking spray

- 2 cups green and red bell pepper, chopped 2 spring onions, chopped

- 1 teaspoon thyme, chopped

- Salt and black pepper to the taste 1 cup coconut cream

- 4 eggs, whisked

- 1 cup cheddar cheese, grated

Directions:

1. In a bowl, mix all the ingredients except the cooking spray and the cheese and whisk well. Grease a pan that fits the air fryer with the cooking spray, pour the bell peppers and eggs mixture, spread, sprinkle the

cheese on top, put the pan in the machine and cook at 350 degrees F for 30 minutes.

2.   Divide between plates and serve for breakfast.

Nutrition: calories 251, fat 16, fiber 3, carbs 6, protein 11

Zucchini Cakes

Prep time: 10 minutes

Cooking time: 8 minutes

Servings: 4

Ingredients:

- 2 zucchini, grated

- 3 tablespoons almond flour

- 1 medium egg, beaten

- ¼ teaspoon salt

- ¼ teaspoon ground black pepper

- ¼ teaspoon minced garlic

- 1 tablespoon spring onions, chopped

- ¼ teaspoon chili flakes

Directions:

1.   Put the grated zucchini in the bowl and add the almond flour. Then add egg, salt, ground black pepper, minced garlic, onion, and chili flakes. Add green peas and

stir the ingredients with the help of the fork until homogenous. Preheat the air fryer to 365F. With the help of the spoon make the fritters and put them on the baking paper. Place the baking paper with fritters in the air fryer and cook them for 4 minutes. Then flip the fritters on another side and cook them for 4 minutes more.

Nutrition: calories 160, fat 11.8, fiber 3.9, carbs 9.6, protein 7.6

Chives Yogurt Eggs

Preparation time: 5 minutes

Cooking time: 20 minutes

Servings: 4

Ingredients:

• Cooking spray

• Salt and black pepper to the taste 1 and ½ cups Greek yogurt

• 4 eggs, whisked

• 1 tablespoon chives, chopped 1 tablespoon cilantro, chopped

Directions:

1. In a bowl, mix all the ingredients except the cooking spray and whisk well. Grease a pan that fits the air fryer with the cooking spray, pour the eggs mix, spread well, put the pan into the machine and cook the omelet at 360 degrees F for 20 minutes. Divide between plates and serve for breakfast.

Nutrition: calories 221, fat 14, fiber 4, carbs 6, protein 11

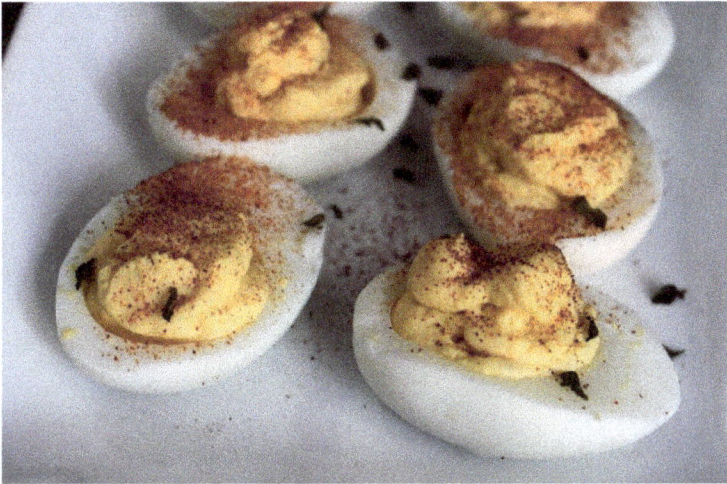

Hot Cups

Prep time: 10 minutes

Cooking time: 3 minutes

Servings: 6

Ingredients:

- 6 eggs, beaten

- 2 jalapeno, sliced

- 2 oz bacon, chopped, cooked

- ½ teaspoon salt

- ½ teaspoon chili powder

- Cooking spray

Directions:

1. Spay the silicone egg molds with cooking spray from inside. In the mixing bowl mix up beaten eggs, sliced jalapeno, salt, bacon, and chili powder.

2. Stir the liquid gently and pour in the egg molds. Preheat the air fryer to 400F. Place the molds with the

egg mixture in the air fryer. Cook the meal for 3 minutes. Then cool the cooked jalapeno & bacon cups for 2-3 minutes and remove from the silicone molds.

Nutrition: calories 116, fat 8.4, fiber 0.2, carbs 0.9, protein 9.1

Green Scramble

Preparation time: 5 minutes

Cooking time: 20 minutes

Servings: 4

Ingredients:

- 1 tablespoon olive oil

- ½ teaspoon smoked paprika 12 eggs, whisked

- 3 cups baby spinach

- Salt and black pepper to the taste

Directions:

1.   In a bowl, mix all the ingredients except the oil and whisk them well. Heat up your air fryer at 360 degrees F, add the oil, heat it up, add the eggs and spinach mix, cover, cook for 20 minutes, divide between plates and serve.

Nutrition: calories 220, fat 11, fiber 3, carbs 4, protein 6

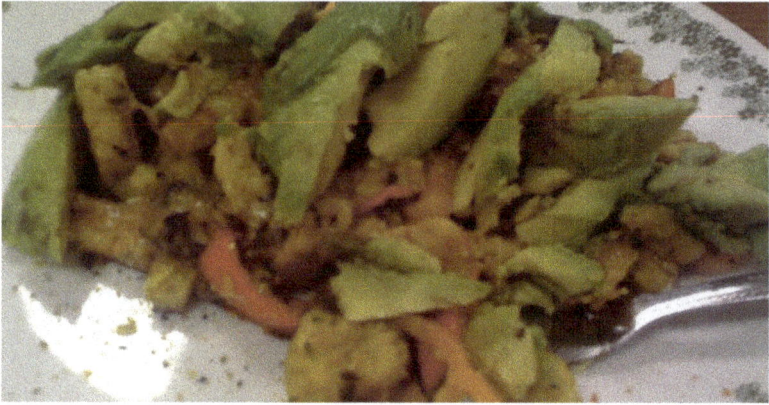

Creamy Veggie Omelet

Prep time: 10 minutes

Cooking time: 14 minutes

Servings: 4

Ingredients:

- 4 eggs, beaten
- 1 tablespoon cream cheese
- ½ teaspoon chili flakes
- ½ cup broccoli florets, chopped
- ¼ teaspoon salt
- ¼ cup heavy cream
- ¼ teaspoon white pepper
- Cooking spray

Directions:

1.   Put the beaten eggs in the big bowl. Add chili flakes, salt, and white pepper. With the help of the hand whisker stir the liquid until the salt is dissolved. Then add

cream cheese and heavy cream. Stir the ingredients until you get the homogenous liquid. After this, add broccoli florets.

2.   Preheat the air fryer to 375F. Spray the air fryer basket with cooking spray from inside. Pour the egg liquid in the air fryer basket. Cook the omelet for 14 minutes.

Nutrition: calories 102, fat 8.1, fiber 0.3, carbs 1.5, protein 6.2

Cheddar Turkey Casserole

Preparation time: 5 minutes

Cooking time: 25 minutes

Servings: 4

Ingredients:

• turkey breast, skinless, boneless, cut into strips and browned 2 teaspoons olive oil

• cups almond milk

• 2 cups cheddar cheese, shredded 2 eggs, whisked

• Salt and black pepper to the taste 1 tablespoon chives, chopped

Directions:

1. In a bowl, mix the eggs with milk, cheese, salt, pepper and the chives and whisk well. Preheat the air fryer at 330 degrees F, add the oil, heat it up, add the turkey pieces and spread them well. Add the eggs mixture, toss a bit and cook for 25 minutes. Serve right away for breakfast.

Nutrition: calories 244, fat 11, fiber 4, carbs 5, protein 7

Spiced Baked Eggs

Prep time: 10 minutes

Cooking time: 3 minutes

Servings: 2

Ingredients:

2 eggs

- 1 teaspoon mascarpone

- ¼ teaspoon ground nutmeg

- ¼ teaspoon dried basil

- ¼ teaspoon dried oregano

- ¼ teaspoon dried cilantro

- ¼ teaspoon ground turmeric

- ¼ teaspoon onion powder

- ¼ teaspoon salt

Directions:

1.   Crack the eggs in the mixing bowl and whisk them well. After this, add mascarpone and stir until you get a

homogenous mixture. Then add all spices and mix up the liquid gently. Pour it in the silicone egg molds and transfer in the air fryer basket. Cook the egg cups for 3 minutes at 400F.

Nutrition: calories 72, fat 4.9, fiber 0.2, carbs 1.1, protein 5.9

Mixed Peppers Hash

Preparation time: 5 minutes

Cooking time: 20 minutes

Servings: 4

Ingredients:

- 1 red bell pepper, cut into strips
- green bell pepper, cut into strips 1 orange bell pepper, cut into strips 4 eggs, whisked
- Salt and black pepper to the taste
- tablespoons mozzarella, shredded cooking spray

Directions:

1. In a bowl, mix the eggs with all the bell peppers, salt and pepper and toss. Preheat the air fryer at 350 degrees F, grease it with cooking spray, pour the eggs mixture, spread well, sprinkle the mozzarella on top and cook for 20 minutes. Divide between plates and serve for breakfast.

Nutrition: calories 229, fat 13, fiber 3, carbs 4, protein 7

Baked Eggs

Prep time: 10 minutes

Cooking time: 10 minutes

Servings: 3

Ingredients:

- 3 eggs

- ½ teaspoon ground turmeric

- ¼ teaspoon salt

- 3 bacon slices

- 1 teaspoon butter, melted

Directions:

1.   Brush the muffin silicone molds with ½ teaspoon of melted butter. Then arrange the bacon in the silicone molds in the shape of circles. Preheat the air fryer to 400F. Cook the bacon for 7 minutes. After this, brush the center of every bacon circle with remaining butter. Then crack the eggs in every bacon circles, sprinkle with salt

and ground turmeric. Cook the bacon cups for 3 minutes more.

Nutrition: calories 178, fat 13.6, fiber 0.1, carbs 0.9, protein 12.6

Paprika Cauliflower Bake

Preparation time: 5 minutes

Cooking time: 20 minutes

Servings: 4

Ingredients:

- 2 cups cauliflower florets, separated 4 eggs, whisked

- teaspoon sweet paprika

- tablespoons butter, melted

- A pinch of salt and black pepper

Directions:

1. Heat up your air fryer at 320 degrees F, grease with the butter, add cauliflower florets on the bottom, then add eggs whisked with paprika, salt and pepper, toss and cook for 20 minutes. Divide between plates and serve for breakfast.

Nutrition: calories 240, fat 9, fiber 2, carbs 4, protein 8

Cinnamon French Toast

Prep time: 12 minutes

Cooking time: 9 minutes

Servings: 2

Ingredients:

- 1/3 cup almond flour

- 1 egg, beaten

- ¼ teaspoon baking powder

- 2 teaspoons Erythritol

- ¼ teaspoon vanilla extract

- 1 teaspoon cream cheese

- ¼ teaspoon ground cinnamon

- 1 teaspoon ghee, melted

Directions:

1.   In the mixing bowl mix up almond flour, baking powder, and ground cinnamon. Then add egg, vanilla extract, ghee, and cream cheese. Stir the mixture with

the help of the fork until homogenous. Line the mugs bottom with baking paper. After this, transfer the almond flour mixture in the mugs and flatten well. Then preheat the air fryer to 355F. Place the mugs with toasts in the air fryer basket and cook them for 9 minutes. When the time is finished and the toasts are cooked, cool them little. Then sprinkle the toasts with Erythritol.

Nutrition: calories 85, fat 7.2, fiber 0.7, carbs 1.8, protein 3.9

Cheddar Tomatoes Hash

Preparation time: 5 minutes

Cooking time: 25 minutes

Servings: 4

Ingredients:

*   2 tablespoons olive oil

*   pound tomatoes, chopped

*   ½ pound cheddar, shredded

*   tablespoons chives, chopped Salt and black pepper to the taste 6 eggs, whisked

Directions:

1.   Add the oil to your air fryer, heat it up at 350 degrees F, add the tomatoes, eggs, salt and pepper and whisk. Also add the cheese on top and sprinkle the chives on top. Cook for 25 minutes, divide between plates and serve for breakfast.

Nutrition: calories 221, fat 8, fiber 3, carbs 4, protein 8

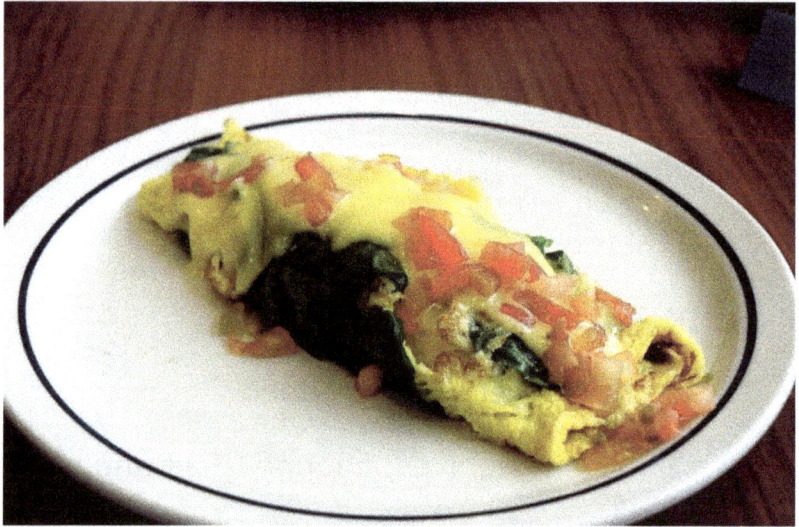

Scotch Eggs

Prep time: 15 minutes

Cooking time: 13 minutes

Servings: 4

Ingredients:

- 4 medium eggs, hard-boiled, peeled

- 9 oz ground beef

- 1 teaspoon garlic powder

- ¼ teaspoon cayenne pepper

- 1 oz coconut flakes

- ¼ teaspoon curry powder

- 1 egg, beaten

- 1 tablespoon almond flour

- Cooking spray

Directions:

1.   In the mixing bowl combine together ground beef and garlic powder. Add cayenne pepper, almond flour,

and curry powder. Stir the meat mixture until homogenous. After this, wrap the peeled eggs in the ground beef mixture. In the end, you should get meat balls. Coat every ball in the beaten egg and then sprinkle with coconut flakes. Preheat the air fryer to 400F. Then spray the air fryer basket with cooking spray and place the meat eggs inside. Cook the eggs for 13 minutes. Carefully flip the scotch eggs on another side after 7 minutes of cooking.

Nutrition: calories 272, fat 16, fiber 1.5, carbs 4.3, protein 28.6

Cheesy Frittata

Preparation time: 10 minutes

Cooking time: 20 minutes

Servings: 6

Ingredients:

- 1 cup almond milk cooking spray

- 9 ounces cream cheese, soft

- 1 cup cheddar cheese, shredded 6 spring onions, chopped

- Salt and black pepper to the taste 6 eggs, whisked

Directions:

1. Heat up your air fryer with the oil at 350 degrees F and grease it with cooking spray. In a bowl, mix the eggs with the rest of the ingredients, whisk well, pour and spread into the air fryer and cook everything for 20 minutes. Divide everything between plates and serve.

Nutrition: calories 231, fat 11, fiber 3, carbs 5, protein 8

Eggs Ramekins

Prep time: 5 minutes

Cooking time: 6 minutes

Servings: 5

Ingredients:

- 5 eggs

- 1 teaspoon coconut oil, melted

- ¼ teaspoon ground black pepper

Directions:

1. Brush the ramekins with coconut oil and crack the eggs inside. Then sprinkle the eggs with ground black pepper and transfer in the air fryer. Cook the baked eggs for 6 minutes at 355F.

Nutrition: calories 144, fat 8, fiber 4.5, carbs 9.1, protein 8.8

Herbed Omelet

Preparation time: 5 minutes

Cooking time: 20 minutes

Servings: 4

Ingredients:

- 10 eggs, whisked

- ½ cup cheddar, shredded

- 2 tablespoons parsley, chopped 2 tablespoons chives, chopped 2 tablespoons basil, chopped Cooking spray

- Salt and black pepper to the taste

Directions:

1. In a bowl, mix the eggs with all the ingredients except the cheese and the cooking spray and whisk well. Preheat the air fryer at 350 degrees F, grease it with the cooking spray, and pour the eggs mixture inside.

2. Sprinkle the cheese on top and cook for 20 minutes. Divide everything between plates and serve.

Nutrition: calories 232, fat 12, fiber 4, carbs 5, protein 7

Chicken Muffins

Prep time: 10 minutes

Cooking time: 10 minutes

Servings: 6

Ingredients:

- 1 cup ground chicken

- 1 cup ground pork

- ½ cup Mozzarella, shredded

- 1 teaspoon dried oregano

- ½ teaspoon salt

- 1 teaspoon ground paprika

- ½ teaspoon white pepper

- 1 tablespoon ghee, melted

- 1 teaspoon dried dill

- 2 tablespoons almond flour

- 1 egg, beaten

Directions:

1.   In the bowl mix up ground chicken, ground pork, dried oregano, salt, ground paprika, white pepper, dried dill, almond flour, and egg. When you get the homogenous texture of the mass, add ½ of all Mozzarella and mix up the mixture gently with the help of the spoon. Then brush the silicone muffin molds with melted ghee. Put the meat mixture in the muffin molds. Flatten the surface of every muffin with the help of the spoon and top with remaining Mozzarella. Preheat the air fryer to 375F. Then arrange the muffins in the air fryer basket and cook them for 10 minutes. Cool the cooked muffins to the room temperature and remove from the muffin molds.

Nutrition: calories 291, fat 20.6, fiber 1.3, carbs 2.7, protein 23.9

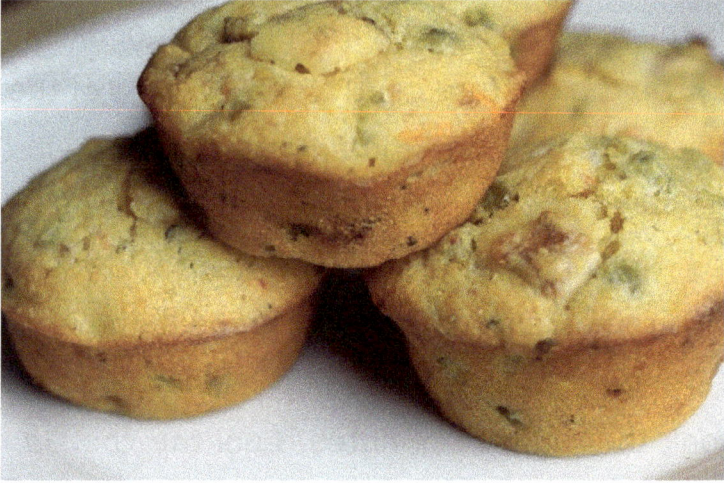

Olives and Eggs Mix

Preparation time: 5 minutes

Cooking time: 20 minutes

Servings: 4

Ingredients:

- 2 cups black olives, pitted and chopped 4 eggs, whisked
- ¼ teaspoon sweet paprika
- 1 tablespoon cilantro, chopped
- ½ cup cheddar, shredded
- A pinch of salt and black pepper Cooking spray

Directions:

1. In a bowl, mix the eggs with the olives and all the ingredients except the cooking spray and stir well. Heat up your air fryer at 350 degrees F, grease it with cooking spray, pour the olives and eggs mixture, spread and cook for 20 minutes. Divide between plates and serve for breakfast.

Nutrition: calories 240, fat 14, fiber 3, carbs 5, protein 8

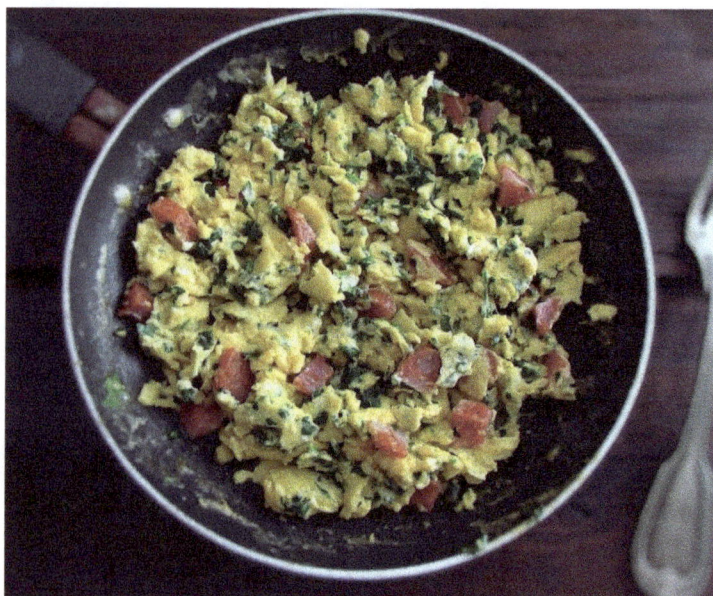

www.ingramcontent.com/pod-product-compliance
Lightning Source LLC
Chambersburg PA
CBHW050751030426
42336CB00012B/1766